An Introduction to,

ESSENTIAL TREMOR

Abdul Qayyum Rana, MD, FRCPC

Director, Parkinson's Clinic of Eastern Toronto

&

Movement Disorders Center

Consultant Neurologist,

Rouge Valley Hospital, Toronto, Canada

iUniverse, Inc.

New York   Bloomington

iUniverse books may be ordered through booksellers or by contacting:

iUniverse
1663 Liberty Drive
Bloomington, IN 47403
www.iuniverse.com
1-800-Authors (1-800-288-4677)

Because of the dynamic nature of the Internet, any Web addresses or
links contained in this book may have changed since publication and
may no longer be valid. The views expressed in this work are solely those
of the author and do not necessarily reflect the views of the publisher,
and the publisher hereby disclaims any responsibility for them.

ISBN: 978-1-4401-9423-8 (sc)
ISBN: 978-1-4401-9424-5 (ebook)

Printed in the United States of America

iUniverse rev. date: 04/26/10

To my Teachers and Colleagues,

Dr. Ali Ghouse
Dr. Arthur Walters
Dr. David Grimes
Dr. Pierre Bourque

Their dedication to teaching served as an inspiration to me.

PREFACE

"Essential Tremor" is the most common movement disorder, which may be mild in severity, and therefore may not come to medical attention in many cases. However, essential tremor is sometimes quite debilitating and may interfere with one's daily activities. Unfortunately there is no cure for essential tremor, but there are many successful treatments, which can be beneficial to many patients. This guide briefly discusses the etiology, pathophysiology, symptoms and different treatments available for this condition.

This guide may be used by medical students, general practitioners and other healthcare professionals. The patients and their family members who want to learn more about this condition may find useful information in this manual as the content of this booklet has been simplified to a great extent. Some of the information in this guide may represent an overview of the work of many experts in this field. Every effort has been made to present correct and up to date information in this handbook, but medicine is a field with ongoing research and developments, therefore readers may use text books for further information if the content of this primer is found to be insufficient.

Most of the information presented in this manual is considered generally accepted practice; however the

I am very grateful to Ashfique Adlul, a life sciences student, who helped in completing this project, Ryhana Dawood for proof reading, as well as other students who assisted during this project. I am thankful to my colleagues Dr. Paul Jensen, Dr. Tilak Mendis and Dr. Emmanuelle Pourcher who reviewed this publication and provided very useful suggestions about each section. I am also thankful to Evelyn Shifflett for drawing all the illustrations for this booklet. I am especially grateful to my father Abdul Shakoor Khan, my brothers Abdul Jabbar and Abdul Wahab khan, my sisters, my friends Dr. Abid Kareem and Dr. Adnan Al-Sarawi for their encouragement in order to complete this work. Lastly I am very thankful to my wife for her input as an internist especially about the section on medical treatments of essential tremor. Suggestions to improve this booklet are welcome and should be forwarded to the author directly.

Abdul Qayyum Rana, MD, FRCPC

TABLE OF CONTENTS

Chapter 1

INTRODUCTION

Tremor is defined as an involuntary rhythmic oscillation of a body part. Essential tremor is the most common movement disorder.

HISTORY:

Movement disorders are neurological conditions, usually obvious by visual observation. For centuries, they have been known in human history because of their ability to attract visual attention. Therefore descriptions of the movement disorders have been found in the ancient literature.

"Charakasamhita", an ancient book compiled by Agnivesha, was written in Sanskrit language in 2500 B.C. and is found at the University of Benares, India. In chapter 20, entitled Vepathu, a comprehensive description of tremors is documented in this text.

Aulus Cornelius Celsus (c25BC-c50AD), a Roman scholar, compiled an encyclopedia entitled "The Eight Books of Medicine" in which he distinguished the fine tremor from a coarse tremor.

In the second century, ancient Greek physician Claudius Galen (130-201 AD) wrote a book on tremor and convulsions. He described the tremor of the hand at rest. He distinguished between the different types of tremors based on their causes and features. He thought that aged individuals developed tremors because of the loss of strength to control movement in their arms. Galen defined tremor as *"an involuntary alternating up and down motion"*

Ibn-Sina (980-1037), an Arabic philosopher, physician and author of Kitab-al-shifa (the book of healing), wrote a chapter on the diseases of nervous system in the "Canon of Medicine". He discussed the *"motor unrest"*, gave descriptions of tremors and prescribed various treatments for these conditions.

The following statement by Leonardo da Vinci (1452-1519) describes the tremor of the hand and head very well. He writes *"How nerves sometimes operate by themselves without any command from soul. This is clearly apparent for you will see paralytics and those who are shivering and benumbed by cold move their trembling parts such as their head and hands without permission of soul, the soul with all its forces can't prevent them from trembling"*.

John Hunter (1728-1793), a prominent Scottish surgeon in 1776 gave a description of Lord L's tremor as *"Lord L's hands are perpetually in motion; he never feels the sensation of them being tired. When he is asleep his hands are perfectly at rest but when he wakes in a little time they begin to move"*. These features are characteristic of the resting tremor of Parkinson's disease and describe the fact that tremor of Parkinson's disease, like most other movement disorders, disappears during sleep.

James Parkinson (1755--1824) was a general practitioner in London, England who in 1817 published an essay on "Shaking Palsy" in which he described six individuals affected with Shaking Palsy. He described this condition as having "*Involuntary tremulous motion, with lessened muscular power, in parts not in action and even when supported, with a propensity to bend the trunk forwards, and to pass from a walking to a running pace, the senses and intellect being uninjured.*" In this statement he described the tremor, bradykinesia, stooping and festination as the characteristics of shaking palsy, which today is known as Parkinson's disease.

Wilhelm von Humboldt (1767-1835), a German scholar from the Prussian kingdom, writes about himself in his letters to a friend dated from 1829 to 1835 "*I am sorry for having written in such an unclear manner, unfortunately only too often I cause people trouble in deciphering my hand writing, I think about this when I am writing but my attention is not always the same and so I become illegible*" then he talks about his hands *trembling* and attributes this to aging.

In 1836, Most described several cases of tremor in a single family.

In 1887, Danna documented within a single pedigree, three families with 45 individuals affected with tremor. Danna described the different body parts which were affected with tremor, severity of tremor, age of onset, absence of tremor during sleep and no effect of tremor on mortality. Danna thought essential tremor was related to neurosis, epilepsy, high intellect and psychosis.

In 1889, Charcot described head tremor in two elderly patients. The tremor he described was rhythmic and was in both horizontal and vertical directions.

In 1909, Raymond related the essential tremor to neuropathic shock, which he thought to be the precipitant of essential tremor.

In 1948, Katzenstein and in the 1920s a Russian neurologist Minor linked essential tremor with longevity.

In 1949, Critchley also thought that essential tremor was linked to high intelligence and accomplishment.

CLASSIFICATION OF TREMOR:

A. *According to the position of the body part affected by tremor*

Tremor is categorized as resting tremor (if the tremor occurs while the affected body part is in complete repose), postural tremor (if the tremor occurs while the affected body part is in steady posture) or kinetic tremor (if the tremor occurs while the affected body part is exerting a movement).

B. *According to the regions of body affected*

Tremor may affect different body parts including limbs, head, tongue, jaw, vocal cords and palate. The parts of the body that are affected by tremor depend upon the underlying neurological condition.

C. *According to the frequency of tremor*

1. Low frequency tremor e.g. tremor of Parkinson's disease
2. Medium frequency tremor e.g. Essential tremor
3. High frequency tremor e.g. Orthostatic tremor

D. *According to the amplitude of tremor*

1. Mild amplitude
2. Moderate amplitude
3. Severe amplitude

E. *According to the etiology of tremor*

1. Essential tremor
2. Enhanced physiological tremor
3. Drug or toxin induced tremor.
4. Dystonic tremor
5. Cerebellar tremor
6. Holmes tremor (mid brain tremor)
7. Primary orthostatic tremor.
8. Cortical tremor
9. Peripheral neuropathy associated tremor.

10. Tremor of Parkinson's disease.
11. Psychogenic tremor
12. Tremor is also seen in many other medical conditions such as thyroid disease, Wilson disease, hypoxia, hypotension, AIDS, hereditary hemochromatosis.
13. Task specific tremor such as primary writing tremor.
14. Post traumatic tremor

As mentioned above, essential tremor is the most common movement disorder.

TERMINOLOGY OF TREMOR:

I. Resting tremor

Resting tremor is evident when the affected body part is in complete repose, supported against gravity and is not voluntarily activated. During the onset of voluntary activity, the tremor completely disappears or the amplitude of the tremor becomes less prominent. Some of the common causes of resting tremor are as follows,

a. Parkinson's disease
b. Parkinson plus syndromes
c. Holmes tremor or Midbrain tremor, which has postural and action components as well.
d. Wilson's disease
e. Essential tremor when severe may have a resting component if limbs not fully relaxed.

II. Action tremor

Action tremor occurs during voluntary activity of the affected body part or when the affected body part is maintaining a steady posture against gravity, and diminishes or completely disappears at rest. This includes postural and kinetic tremors.

a. *Postural tremor*

This subtype of action tremor occurs when the affected body part is voluntarily supporting itself against gravity.

b. *Kinetic tremor*

This subtype of action tremor occurs when the affected body part is performing a voluntary activity which could be goal directed or non goal directed.

Some of the examples of action tremor are as follows,

a. Enhanced physiological tremor
   i) anxiety or emotional stress.
   ii) endocrine: hypoglycemia, thyrotoxicosis, pheochromocytoma, adrenocorticosteroids
   iii) drugs and toxins: beta agonists, amphetamines, theophylline, caffeine and alcohol withdrawal etc
b. Essential tremor
c. Primary writing tremor
d. Other neurological conditions such as,
   i) Parkinson's disease when resting tremor is severe

ii) Parkinson plus syndromes especially multiple system atrophy

iii) dystonic tremor including idiopathic focal dystonias

e. Peripheral neuropathy

f. Cerebellar tremor

III. Intention tremor

This type of tremor is present if the amplitude of the tremor increases when the affected body part is approaching the target. This is seen with cerebellar pathology.

IV. Task-specific kinetic tremor

This type of tremor occurs during a specific activity such as primary writing tremor.

DESCRIPTION OF TREMOR:

The following parameters should be included when describing a particular tremor:

1. Topography (eg: head, limbs, chin, jaw, etc.)
2. The position of affected body part in which tremor is most prominent (eg: rest, postural, activity, specific task)
3. The frequency of the tremor
4. The amplitude of tremor

Tremor Syndrome	Frequency HZ
Enhanced physiological tremor	10-14
Essential tremor syndrome	7-10
Primary orthostatic tremor	14-18
Task specific tremor	4-8
Holmes tremor	3-5
Tremor of Parkinson's disease	3-7
Cerebellar tremor	3-5
Palatal tremor	2-6
Dystonic tremor	5-7
Alcoholic tremor	3-4
Toxic and drug induced tremor	5-10
Psychogenic tremor	Variable

Table 1.1 Frequencies of Different Tremor Syndromes

REFERENCES:

Bendick, J., Galen and the Gateway to Medicine, Bethelem Books, Bathgate, ND 2000

Broussolle E., Krack P., Thobois S., Xie-Brustolin J., Pollak P., Goetz C.G., Movement Disorders 2007;2: 223-236 "An Essay on the Shaking Palsy" James Parkinson

Elble R.J., Characteristics of physiologic tremor in young and elderly adults. Clin Neurophysiol 2003;114:624-35.

Elble R.J. Essential Tremor; Medlink, February 2007

Guillain, G., J.M. Charcot, 1825-1893, His Life — His Work; New York, NY: Paul B. Hoeber, 1959

Horowski R., Horowski L., Vogel S., Poewe W., Kielhorn F.W., An essay on Wilhelm von Humboldt and the shaking palsy. Neurology 1995; 45 part 1: 565-568

Jankovic J.,Tolosa E., Parkinson's Disease and Movement Disorders. Fifth edition, Lippincott Philadelphia, PA 2007

Kim Y.J., Pakiam A.S., Lang A.E., Historical and Clinical features of Psychogenic Tremor: a review of 70 cases. Can J of Neurological Sciences 1999;26:190-5.

Leehey M.A., Hagerman R.J., Landau W.M., et al. Tremor/ataxia syndrome in fragile X carrier males. Movement Disorders 2002;17:744-5.

Morris, AD., James Parkinson, His life and times, Boston, MA Reprinted 1989

Online biography of Ibn-e-Sina.en. wikipedia.org

O'Suilleabhain PE, Matsumoto JY. Time-frequency analysis of Tremors. Brain 1998;121:2127-34

Viartis, History of Parkinson's disease. http://viartis. net/parkinsons.disease/history.htm

Chapter 2

CLINICAL FEATURES OF ESSENTIAL TREMOR

EPIDEMIOLOGY:

Essential tremor affects about 5 to 6 percent of the individuals over the age of 65. About 5 to 15 percent of essential tremor cases occur during childhood. Essential tremor may be familial in cases that begin before the age of 20. Essential tremor is common in all races across the world.

The prevalence of essential tremor is significantly higher in individuals above the age of 40. In some studies the prevalence of essential tremor in patients above the age of 40 has been reported to be as high as 10 percent, however, the peak age of onset for essential tremor is 70 to 79 years. The prevalence of essential tremor is 10 times greater in 70 to 79 years old individuals as compared to 40 to 69 years old individuals. Some studies have reported a slightly higher prevalence in men, but other studies could not find any difference between men and women.

There is no effect of essential tremor on life expectancy. A similar survival rate has been reported among patients with essential tremor and their age and sex matched controls. The likelihood of patients with essential tremor having first degree relatives with essential tremor is five times greater than the normal population. There seems to be an increase in prevalence of essential tremor with age. It is estimated that almost 5 million people in the United States, over the age of 40, are affected with essential tremor. Essential tremor is more common than Parkinson's disease.

ONSET:

Essential tremor usually affects both sides of the body, although initially it may only be noticed on one side. It can occur at any age. Although, it may be seen in the early twenties, late onset, after the age of 55 years is more common. Essential tremor may begin in early childhood but its prevalence and intensity increase with advancing age and eventually, it may interfere with writing, eating and other activities of daily life. In familial cases the onset of essential tremor may be much earlier than sporadic cases.

COURSE:

Essential tremor is a slowly progressive condition in which the amplitude of tremor usually increases with time. In some cases there may be no change noted in the tremor for several years, and then in advanced age, the tremor may get worse relatively quickly. In addition, as the amplitude of tremor increases, the frequency of tremor may decrease.

EXACERBATING FACTORS:

Fatigue, central nervous system stimulation, sexual arousal, emotional excitement and temperature extremes can exacerbate the tremor. Alcohol may dampen the tremor significantly. The effect of alcohol seems to be centrally mediated. Caffeine on the other hand, seems to precipitate essential tremor. Essential tremor, like most other movement disorders, disappears in sleep.

ETIOLOGY AND PATHOGENSIS:

The exact cause of essential tremor is unknown. Some patients may have a family history of tremor in their parents, siblings or close relatives. However, sporadic cases are seen quite frequently. The exact mechanism of inheritance is unclear. The terms like "Familial Essential Tremor" and "Benign Essential Tremor" have also been used for essential tremor in literature. The term "Benign Essential Tremor" is misleading as the essential tremor may be quite disabling. In a significant number of cases, essential tremor is hereditary and is transmitted in an autosomal dominant pattern. Chromosome 3q13 and chromosome 2p22-p25 have been suggested to be the disease loci in many reports. Environmental factors may also play a role in the causation of essential tremor. This is supported by the lack of a complete concordance of essential tremor in monozygotic twins.

There is a lack of clear understanding of the pathophysiological mechanisms of essential tremor.

The central nervous system pathology is supported by the observation of response of tremor to thalamotomy and centrally acting drugs. Cerebellum may play an important role in pathophysiology of essential tremor. It is believed that essential tremor may emerge from abnormal oscillations within thalamocortical and cerebello-olivary loops in the brain. This theory is supported by the findings that the lesions or injury of the cerebellar and thalamic regions reduces the intensity of essential tremor. Neuronal discharges correlated to tremor have been observed to occur in the ventrolateral thalamus, particularly in the ventralis intermedius nucleus. Contralateral limb tremor can be suppressed by the ablation or high frequency stimulation of ventralis intermedius nucleus of thalamus. Essential tremor may be the result of abnormal oscillations of a central nervous system pacemaker. This central oscillator could be enhanced or suppressed, however the exact location of this oscillator is unknown.

GENERAL PRESENTATION:

The patients usually complain of their handwriting becoming sloppy and large, trouble holding objects like a cup of coffee, using fork, spoon, keys, screwdriver and pouring liquids. They may spill liquids and writing a cheque may be a challenge. In severe cases essential tremor may interfere with dressing, preparing meals and other activities of daily living. Essential tremor is temporarily dampened by intake of alcohol. The history of response to alcohol is helpful diagnostically.

Examiner   Patient

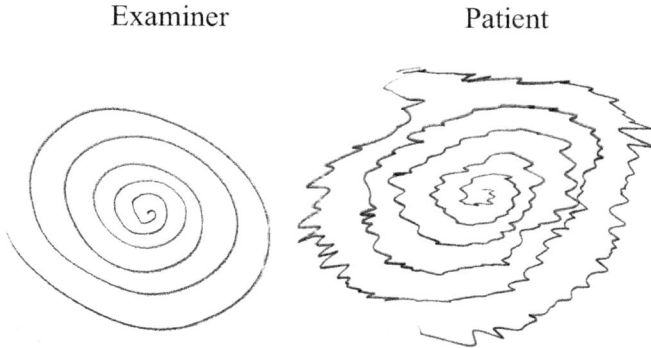

Figure 2.1 Spiral drawing by the examiner and
a patient with Essential Tremor (Spiral Test)

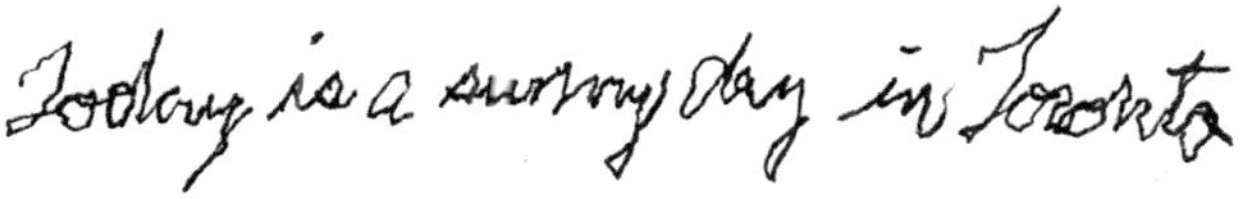

(Today is a sunny day in Toronto)

Figure 2.2 Hand writing of a patient
with very mild Essential Tremor

The pediatric cases of essential tremor affect more
males than females. Most patients with essential tremor
seek attention only if they have a functional or social
disability because of tremor. Essential tremor may
result in social phobia due to embarrassment.

Patients with essential tremor may have mild neuro-
psychological deficits, including problems with
visual perception, encoding, and verbal fluency as
well as working memory. One population-based

study suggested that the older individuals with essential tremor are almost twice as likely to have dementia when compared with the age matched individuals without essential tremor, in addition, that the essential tremor is associated with about a 60% increased risk of developing dementia. This study indicated that the prevalence of dementia among patients with essential tremor is beyond what is expected with age associated cognitive decline, and suggested that the physicians should be discussing the cognitive issues as well as possible treatment options with these elderly patients with essential tremor. The average age of patients included in this study was 77 years. Although, the exact cause of increased risk for dementia among the essential tremor patients remains unknown. However, this study did not include younger patients with essential tremor. No relation between MCI (mild cognitive impairment) and essential tremor was found, although most MCI patients ultimately develop dementia.

Classical essential tremor is a monosymptomatic, postural and action tremor. Essential tremor usually affects the upper extremities and the hands, but it may also involve the head, lower extremities, voice and other body parts. In classic essential tremor the approximate frequency of involvement of different body parts is as follows,

Region of body	Frequency
Hands and arms	90-95 %
Head	30-35 %
Tongue	25-30 %
Legs	25-30 %
Voice	10-15 %
Face and Jaw	7%
Trunk	5%

Table 2.1 Approximate frequency of involvement of different body regions in Essential tremor

CHARACTERISTICS OF TREMOR:

Essential tremor is only present when the affected body part is exerting effort and not during repose. Mental tasks or stress may exacerbate the essential tremor. Essential tremor does not occur during sleep, but patients sometimes complain of an especially coarse tremor upon awakening in the morning.

Essential tremor affecting the hands causes a flexion extension movement of the hands, abduction movement of the fingers and, only in minority of cases, supination-pronation movements of the hands or arms. The size of handwriting is usually large (macrographia) in contrast to the tremor of Parkinson's disease, in which the size of handwriting is small (micrographia). The legs, tongue, voice, face and trunk if involved in essential tremor, are usually affected in the later stages of the disease.

17

The tremor of the hands is usually of medium frequency in the range of 7-10 Hz. It becomes more apparent with arms outstretched, extended or straight at elbows with fingers apart, as well as with arms outstretched, flexed at elbows in front of the chest with fingers apart (wing beating position) and during the finger-nose-finger movements.

The frequency of tremor varies with age, severity and the location in the body. The tremor frequency usually slows down with age, at a rate of about 0.07Hz per year. This decrease in frequency causes a gradual increase in tremor amplitude over the years. Patients with severe essential tremor may also have difficulty with tandem gait which is tested by walking heel-to-toe. Neurological examination is otherwise normal.

Essential tremor in the upper limbs is usually symmetric or only mildly asymmetric. Women with essential tremor are more likely to develop a head tremor. The presence of only unilateral tremor usually indicates the presence of other conditions, like early Parkinson's disease, focal dystonia or primary writing tremor. Advanced essential tremor may show crescendo accentuation as the hand approaches its target, resembling cerebellar intention tremor. No definite evidence indicating a relationship between essential tremor and other neurological conditions has been found. Essential tremor is a syndrome that is defined clinically and thus it is not a specific disease.

A *jaw tremor* can occur in both essential tremor and in Parkinson's disease. It is the presence of other clinical features along with the jaw tremor that indicates which of two conditions is present. Essential tremor involving the jaw tends to occur in patients with head tremor, voice tremor, and more severe upper extremities tremor. On the other hand, the presence of jaw tremor and resting tremor in the absence of action tremor in the hands, voice or head tremor would lead one to suspect Parkinson's disease.

VARIANTS OF ESSENTIAL TREMOR:

Isolated Head Tremor:

Isolated head tremor may be a variant of essential tremor or dystonic in nature. In the case of essential tremor variant, some patients with isolated head tremor may develop limb tremor even years after the onset of the head tremor. Isolated head tremor, without limb tremor, should be carefully differentiated from dystonic tremor. Patients with dystonic tremor may give a history of their neck being pulled or turned to one side or the other. On examination, their head may be turned, tilted or shifted to one side or the other, and there may be asymmetry in the size of the head and neck muscles. History of sensory tricks indicates dystonic tremor. However, some workers strongly feel that isolated head tremor (i.e. without limb tremor) is most often a form of cervical dystonia.

Isolated Tongue Tremor:

Isolated tongue tremor is infrequent. Affected patients may be unaware of any tremor involving their tongue. Tongue tremor may affect speaking, as well as eating.

Isolated Voice Tremor:

Isolated voice tremor is only limited to the voice. It has two types: a pure voice tremor, which is considered a form of essential tremor, and a second type with a dysphonic voice which is similar to spasmodic dysphonia. The latter type is considered to be a form of focal dystonia of the vocal cords. Voice tremor may occur in cerebellar disease but does not fit with the definition of isolated voice tremor because it usually has the other cerebellar features accompanied with the voice tremor. Dystonic voice tremor can often be successfully treated with botulinum toxin injections in to the vocal cords which may also be helpful in the essential tremor variant of voice tremor. Thalamic deep-brain stimulation may reduce voice tremor. Essential tremor may involve speech; however, isolated essential tremor affecting speech may be difficult to differentiate from a dystonic tremor.

Isolated Facial Tremor:

Isolated facial tremor is also an essential tremor variant, however, it is rare. Isolated facial tremor is apparent with half-hearted smile, and may be mistaken for bilateral hemifacial spasm or synkinesis due to Bells Palsy.

Isolated Trunk Tremor:

Essential tremor affecting the trunk is very rare. These patients may have a long history of severe arm and head tremor.

Isolated Chin Tremor:

This rare type of high frequency tremor involves the mentalis muscle of the chin. This type of tremor typically starts in early childhood and is an autosomal dominant hereditary condition. A low frequency chin tremor is also seen in Parkinson's disease, but the other features of Parkinson's disease are more obvious in these patients.

Primary Writing Tremor and other Task or Position Specific Tremors:

This type of tremor involves the highly skilled professional activities, and the more common daily motor activities or movements such as eating, drinking fluids or handling other objects are not affected. Patients who usually suffer from this type of tremor are those who perform motor activities at the highest level, such as musicians or sportsmen. It is controversial whether task specific tremor is a variant of essential tremor or dystonic tremor. Task specific writing tremor is one of the most common task specific tremor. *Task specific writing tremor type A* occurs only during the act of writing, while the *task specific writing tremor type B* occurs even when the hand assumes the writing position.

REFERENCES:

Bain PG, Findley LJ, Thompson PD, et al. A study of hereditary essential tremor. Brain 1994;117:805-24.

Benito-Leon J, Louis ED, Bermejo-Pareja F. Population-based case-control study of cognitive function in essential tremor. Neurology 2006;66:69-74.

Berry-Kravis E, Lewin F, Wuu J, et al. Tremor and ataxia in fragile X premutation carriers: blinded videotape study. Annals of Neurology 2003;53:616-23.

Bradley GW., Daroff R., Fenichel G., Marsden D. Neurology in Clinical Practice, Third edition. Butterworth & Heinmann, Woburn, MA 2000

Brin MF, Koller W. Epidemiology and genetics of essential tremor. Movement Disorders 2000;13(Supplement 3):55-63.

Busenbark KL, Nash J, Nash S, Hubble JP, Koller WC. Is essential tremor benign? Neurology 1991;41:1982-3

Cooper C, Evidente VG, Hentz JG, Adler CH, Caviness JN, Gwinn-Hardy K. The effect of temperature on hand function in patients with tremor. J Hand Ther 2000;13:276-88.

Deuschl G, Elble RJ. The Pathophysiology of Essential Tremor. Neurology 2000;54:S14-20.

Elble RJ. Essential tremor frequency decreases with time. Neurology 2000b;55:1547-51.

Elble RJ. Essential tremor is a monosymptomatic disorder. Movement Disorders 2002;17:633-7.

Elble RJ. Essential Tremor: Medlink. February 2007

Elble RJ. Report from a U.S. conference on essential tremor. Movement Disorders 2006;21:2052-61.

Elble RJ. The role of aging in the clinical expression of essential tremor. Exp Gerontol 1995;30:337-47.

Gasparini M, Bonifati V, Fabrizio E, et al. Frontal lobe dysfunction in essential tremor: a preliminary study. J Neurol 2001;248:399-402.

Goetz, CG. Textbook of Clinical Neurology, second edition, Saunders, Philadelphia, PA 2003

Gulcher JR, Jonsson P, Kong A, et al. Mapping of a familial essential tremor gene, FET1, to chromosome 3q13. Nat Genet 1997;17:84-7.

Hardesty DE, Maragancre DM, Matsumoto JY, Louis ED. Increased risk of head tremor in women with essential tremor: longitudinal data from the Rochester Epidemiology Project. Movement Disorders 2004;19:529-33.

Hellwig B, Häussler S, Schelter B, et al. Tremor-correlated cortical activity in essential tremor. Lancet 2001;357:519-23

Helmchen C, Hagenow A, Miesner J, et al. Eye movement abnormalities in essential tremor may indicate cerebellar dysfunction. Brain 2003;126:1319-32.

Higgins JJ, Lombardi RQ, Pucilowska J, Jankovic J, Tan EK, Rooney JP. A variant in the HS1-BP3 gene is associated with familial essential tremor. Neurology 2005;64(3):417-21.

Higgins JJ, Lombardi RQ, Pucilowska J, Jankovic J, Golbe LI, Verhagen L. HS1-BP3 gene variant is common in familial essential tremor. Movement Disorders 2006;21:306-9.

Higgins JJ, Pho LT, Nee LE. A gene (ETM) for essential tremor maps to chromosome 2p22-p25. Movement Disorders 1997;6:859-64.

Hsu YD, Chang MK, Sung SC, Hsein HH, Deng JC. Essential tremor: clinical, electromyographical and pharmacological studies in 146 Chinese patients. Chung Hua I Hsueh Tsa Chih (Taipei) 1990;45:93-9.

Hua SE, Lenz FA. Posture-related oscillations in human cerebellar thalamus in essential tremor are enabled by voluntary motor circuits. J Neurophysiol 2005;93:117-27.

Jankovic J. Essential tremor: a heterogenous disorder. Movement Disorders 2002;17:638-44.

Jankovic J.,Tolosa E. Parkinson's Disease and Movement Disorder. Fifth edition, Lippincott Philadelphia, PA 2007

Koster B, Deuschl G, Lauk M, Timmer J, Guschlbauer B, Lücking CH. Essential tremor and cerebellar dysfunction: abnormal ballistic movements. Journal of Neurology, Neurosurgery and Psychiatry 2002;73:400-5.

Kovach MJ, Ruiz J, Kimonis K, et al. Genetic heterogeneity in autosomal dominant Essential Tremor. Genet Med 2001;3:197-9.

Lombardi WJ, Woolston DJ, Roberts JW, Gross RE. Cognitive deficits in patients with essential tremor. Neurology 2001;57:785-90.

Lorenz D, Frederiksen H, Moises H, Kopper F, Deuschl G, Christensen K. High concordance for essential tremor in monozygotic twins of old age. Neurology 2004;62:208-11.

Louis ED, Dure LS, Pullman S. Essential tremor in childhood: a series of nineteen cases. Movement Disorders 2001a;16:921-3.

Louis ED. Etiology of essential tremor: should we be searching for environmental causes? Movement Disorders 2001;16:822-9.

Louis ED, Fernandez-Alvarez E, Dure LS 4th, Frucht S, Ford B. Association between male gender and pediatric essential tremor. Movement Disorders 2005;20:904-6.

Louis ED, Ford B, Frucht S, Barnes LF, Tang MX, Ottman R. Risk of tremor and impairment from tremor in relatives of patients with essential tremor: a community-based family study. Annals of Neurology 2001b;49:761-9.

Louis ED, Ford B, Pullman S, Baron K. How normal is 'normal'? Mild tremor in a multiethnic cohort of normal subjects. Archives of Neurology 1998b;55:222-7.

Louis ED, Ottman R. Study of possible factors associated with age of onset in essential tremor. Movement Disorders 2006;21:1980-6.

Louis ED, Ottman R, Hauser WA. How common is the most common adult movement disorder? Estimates of the prevalence of essential tremor throughout the world. Movement Disorders 1998c;13:5-10.

Louis ED, Rios E, Applegate LM, Hernandez NC, Andrews HF. Jaw tremor: prevalence and clinical correlates in three essential tremor case samples. Movement Disorders 2006c;21:1872-8.

Louis ED, Vonsattel JP, Honig LS, et al. Neuropathologic findings in essential tremor. Neurology 2006a;66:1756-9.

Louis ED, Vonsattel JP, Honig LS, et al. Essential tremor associated with pathologic changes in the cerebellum. Archives of Neurology 2006b;63:1189-93.

Louis ED, Vonsattel JP, Honig LS, et al. Neuropathologic findings in essential tremor. Neurology 2006a;66:1756-9

Louis ED, Wendt KJ, Ford B. Senile tremor: what is the prevalence and severity of tremor in older adults? Gerontology 2000b;46:12-6.

Louis ED, Wendt KJ, Pullman SL, Ford B. Is essential tremor symmetric? Observational data from a community-based study of essential tremor. Archives of Neurology 1998d;55:1553-9.

Ma S, Davis TL, Blair MA, et al. Familial essential tremor with apparent autosomal dominant inheritance: should we also consider other inheritance modes? Movement Disorders 2006;2:1368-74.

Pellecchia MT, Varrone A, Annesi G, et al. Parkinsonism and essential tremor in a family with pseudo-dominant inheritance of PARK2: An FP-CIT SPECT study. Movement Disorders 2006.

Rajput A, Robinson CA, Rajput AH. Essential tremor course and disability: a clinicopathologic study of 20 cases. Neurology 2004;62:932-6.

Ray L.W and Koller W.C. Movement Disorders, Neurologic Principles and Practice. Second edition. McGraw-Hill, USA, 2003.

Sahin HA, Terzi M, Ucak S, Yapici O, Basoglu T, Onar M. Frontal functions in young patients with essential tremor: a case comparison study. J Neuropsychiatry Clin Neurosci 2006;18:64-72.

Shatunov A, Jankovic J, Elble R, et al. A variant in the HS1-BP3 gene is associated with familial essential tremor. Neurology 2005;65(12):1995.

Stolze H, Petersen G, Raethjen J, Wenzelburger R, Deuschl G. The gait disorder of advanced essential tremor. Brain 2001;124:2278-86.

Tan EK, Lum SY, Prakash KM. Clinical features of childhood onset essential tremor. Eur J Neurol 2006;13:1302-5.

Tan EK, Zhao Y, Puong KY, et al. Fragile X premutation alleles in SCA, ET, and Parkinsonism in an Asian cohort. Neurology 2004;63:362-3

Tanner CM, Goldman SM. Lyons KE, et al. Essential tremor in twins: an assessment of genetic versus environmental determinants of etiology. Neurology 2001;57:1389-91.

Thawani S., Schupf N., Louis E. Essential tremor is associated with dementia: Prospective population-based study in New York. Neurology 2009; 73: 621-625.

Chapter 3

DIAGNOSIS OF ESSENTIAL TREMOR

The diagnosis of essential tremor is made by history and physical examination. The CT and MRI scans are normal or may show age related atrophy and are usually not required in typical cases. There are no confirmatory tests for essential tremor.

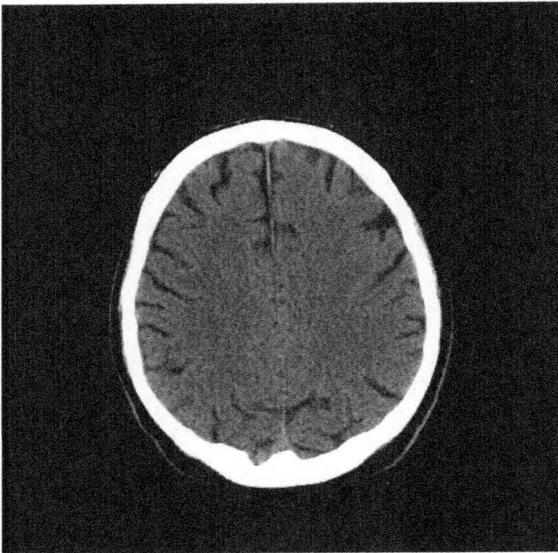

Figure 3.1 CT scan of a 67 year old male with essential tremor

PHYSICAL EXAMINATION:

In addition to a general screening neurological examination, the following steps are helpful in the assessment of essential tremor.

1. Asking the patient to hold arms straight out-stretched, extended at elbows with fingers spread apart.

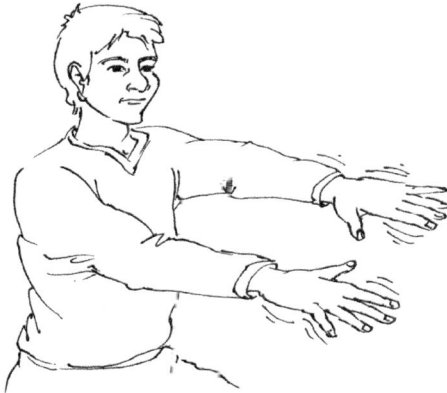

Figure 3.2 Outstretched position
of hands in postural tremor.

2. Holding arms with fingers spread apart, flexed at elbows in front of the chest (wing beating position).

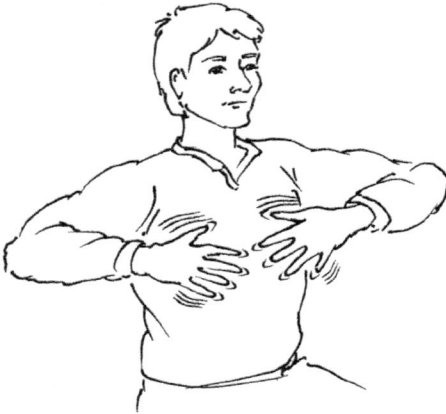

Figure 3.3 Wing beating position
of hands in postural tremor.

3. While arms in the wing beating position, asking
    the patient to make a fist with both hands while
    leaving the index finger of each hand extended,
    pointing towards each other in close proximity
    without touching (author calls this "One to One
    test"). This helps to assess the subtle cases of
    postural tremor.

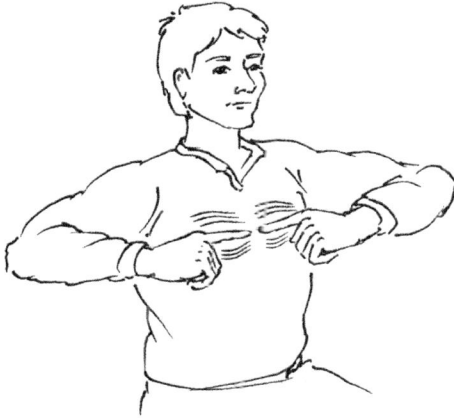

Figure 3.4 One to One Test

4.   Finger-Nose-Finger testing.

5.   Asking the patient to hold a cup, at least four inches
     tall, full of water (up to one inch from the top) and
     to bring it to their lips and then away from their
     mouth a few times to see if there is any spillage of
     water (glass test). Pouring of liquids may also be
     tested.

6.   Writing a standard sentence on each visit. The
     author asks the patients to write *"Today is a sunny
     day in Toronto"* on each visit. The new writing
     sample on each visit is then compared to the
     writing sample from the previous visit in order to
     assess the therapeutic response.

7.   Drawing a spiral without supporting the hand on
     the clipboard on each visit and comparing the

drawing to the one from previous visit in order to assess the therapeutic response.

8. Examining for facial tremor in the half- hearted smile.

9. Determining the involvement of the voice by sustained phonation and asking the patient to hold a prolonged note such as "EEEEEEEEEEEE" as well as conversation.

10. Inspecting the head carefully for tremor as well as for any abnormal position, such as a turn or tilt to any side, anterocollis (forward bending) or retrocollis (backward bending) and sagittal or lateral shift of head which may be seen in a dystonic tremor. The author finds it helpful to inspect the patient from front, behind as well as from each side, standing at a distance of 6-9 feet from the patient to determine the abnormal head or neck position. Mild head tremor may be easily missed unless the head is examined in different positions, both vertically and horizontally. The author usually asks patients to close their eyes for a few minutes, relax and let their head do what it likes to do without any active movement. Neck muscles should be inspected and palpated for any asymmetry in size if the dystonic tremor is suspected.

11. The tongue is examined at rest in the mouth and while it is partially protruded out.

12. Lips, jaw, chin and lower extremities should also

be examined for tremor. Tremor in the legs can be assessed by flexion at hips and knees with foot in dorsi-flexion.

13. To assess the features of parkinsonism, the following examination is conducted:

a. Examination for resting tremor with hands, arms and legs at complete rest supported against gravity in supine position.

b. Examination for rigidity, which is a velocity independent increase in muscle tone, by passive movements at wrists and elbows. A mild cogwheeling of upper extremities may be present in many elderly individuals but is not significant when other features of parkinsonism are absent.

c. Examination for bradykinesia by fist clenching, finger tapping, rapid supination and pronation of arms and leg agility movements. Decrease in speed, drop in amplitude or early fatigue is a sign of bradykinesia.

d. Examination of gait including ability to stand up from a deep seated chair, start hesitation, base and speed of walking, stride length, arm swing, posture of trunk and turning should be observed carefully. Gait should also be observed for any freezing, which is the sudden cessation of mobility while walking. Freezing may occur at the start of walking, going through the doorway, turning or reaching the destination. Freezing may be seen in parkinsonism and is more common in atypical parkinsonism.

e. Pull test for assessment of postural reflexes.

14. To assess cerebellar involvement, the following examination is conducted:

a. Assessment for dysdiadokinesia.

b. Heel-Knee-Shin testing.

c. Assessment of speech for dysarthria and examination of extraocular movements for nystagmus. Patients with cerebellar disorders may have scanning of speech and rebound nystagmus.

Before making a final diagnosis, the other causes of tremor such as medications (lithium, valproic acid, thyroxin, antipsychotics etc), anxiety, hyperthyroidism, task specific writing tremor, and focal neurological abnormalities should be carefully excluded.

CRITERIA FOR THE DIAGNOSIS OF ESSENTIAL TREMOR:

The criteria for the diagnosis of essential tremor includes the presence of a postural tremor in the upper extremities that worsens with action in the absence of other medical conditions or drugs which enhance physiological tremor, cerebellar signs, Parkinson's disease, dystonia, hyperthyroidism, anxiety, peripheral neuropathy and alcoholism.

OR

The postural tremor of the arms without an action component plus a head tremor in the absence of any drugs or medical conditions which enhance the physiological tremor, cerebellar signs, Parkinson's disease and dystonia.

While considering the diagnosis of essential tremor, the primary inclusion features are as follows;

1.) Postural or kinetic tremor of both upper extremities.
2.) Isolated head tremor without any dystonic features.
3.) Absence of other focal findings except mild cogwheeling especially in the elderly patients.

The secondary inclusion features are as follows;

1.) Long duration (more than three years)
2.) Family history of essential tremor
3.) Responsiveness to alcohol

The features suggesting exclusion of essential tremor are;

1.) Abnormal focal neurological findings or sensory or motor signs
2.) History of recent trauma before the onset of tremor
3.) History of factors that may cause enhanced physiologic tremor
4.) History of presence of psychogenic tremor
5.) History of sudden onset of tremor
6.) History of stepwise progression of tremor
7.) Primary orthostatic tremor
8.) Isolated position-specific or task specific tremor.

9.) Unilateral tremor of prolonged duration, unilateral leg tremor, gait dysfunction, resting tremor, bradykinesia or rigidity.
10.) History of antipsychotics or other drug use that might cause or exacerbate tremor
11.) Isolated head tremor with abnormal posture of head and neck.

DIFFERENTIAL DIAGNOSIS:

Elderly individuals with new onset essential tremor may be misdiagnosed with Parkinson's disease, especially if they have mild cogwheeling at their wrists or elbows, and may be slightly slow in performing the repetitive movements due to their age. The action tremor in these patients may have a slight resting component as well, which is actually a severe postural and kinetic tremor that does not abolish completely in the resting position because of incomplete muscle relaxation. Therefore patients should be examined in recumbent position with complete body support against gravity. Cogwheeling in these cases may be a function of tremor rather than the rigidity associated with Parkinson's disease.

Other conditions which may be mistaken for essential tremor include drug and toxin-induced tremor, cortical tremor, cerebellar outflow tremor, tardive tremor, focal dystonia, tremor associated with severe neuropathy, posttraumatic tremor, enhanced physiological tremor, psychogenic tremor and a severe Parkinson's disease tremor which may have postural and action components.

Enhanced Physiological tremor is a result of the interaction of numerous mechanical and neuromuscular influences. This type of tremor can be enhanced in amplitude by various psychological and metabolic aggravating factors which include anxiety, fatigue, alcohol withdrawal and hyperthyroidism. Caffeine can also enhance this type of tremor. This tremor has a frequency of 10-14 Hz.

Parkinson's disease tremor is classically a resting tremor that is present when the affected body part is in repose, and diminishes with activity and posture. The frequency of the tremor of Parkinson's disease is low, in the range of 3-7 HZ. It is usually of supination-pronation type and starts on one side of the body, mostly in the hand or arm. It is also called pill rolling tremor. The tremor may start asymmetrically in the thumb or index finger and may involve the hands, arms, legs, and lips but usually does not involve the head or voice. This type of tremor may be accompanied by other signs of Parkinson's disease such as bradykinesia, rigidity and postural instability. History of the other features of Parkinson's disease such as drooling, difficulty with dexterity and micrographia may be elicited.

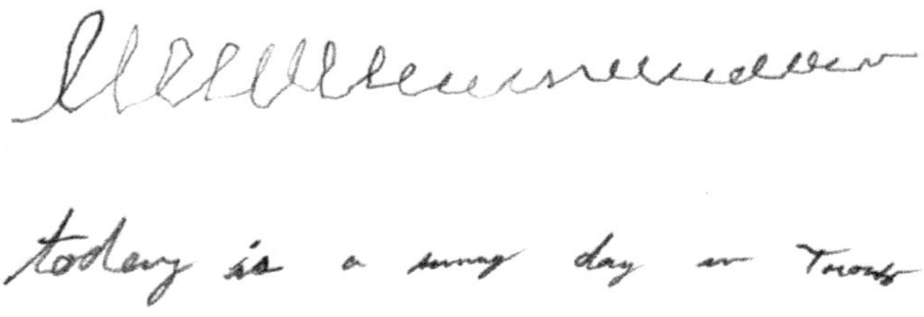

(Today is a sunny day in Toronto)

Figure 3.5 Multiple loops and Handwriting of a Parkinson's disease patient with micrographia.

About 40 percent of the patients with Parkinson's disease may have postural and action tremor in addition to the typical resting tremor of Parkinson's disease. Postural and action tremor may occur in isolation or in combination with resting tremor in Parkinson's disease. Patients with pure resting tremor experience greater social embarrassment than functional disability. Some patients complain of the sensation of trembling inside their body long before a resting tremor becomes apparent. On the other hand, in some cases, it is a family member or a friend who notices the tremor much before it becomes noticeable to the patient. In the face, resting tremor actually affects the lips and jaw and the patient may notice a rhythmic clicking of the teeth.

The prominent head tremor is rarely caused by Parkinson's disease. The severe limb tremor of Parkinson's disease may be conducted to the trunk and head. The tremor in the legs, especially in the feet, while sitting is usually due to Parkinson's disease. Many patients find that they can hide their tremor effectively at will through various methods, such as holding one hand with the other, sitting on the affected hand or crossing the legs to dampen the leg tremor.

Essential tremor usually appears without any latency when the arms are outstretched, while the tremor of Parkinson's disease appears after a latency of at least several seconds when the arms are outstretched from the resting position.

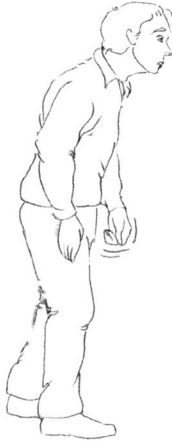

Figure 3.6 Stooping of posture in Parkinson's disease.

The relationship of essential tremor and Parkinson's disease is controversial. Most recent studies conclude that essential tremor and Parkinson's disease are genetically independent conditions. However, some reports in the past have suggested an increased incidence of Parkinson's disease in families of patients with essential tremor and vice versa. About 15-20 percent of patients with essential tremor may be misdiagnosed as Parkinson's disease.

	Enhanced Physiological tremor	Essential tremor	Tremor of Parkinson's disease
Body part affected	Hands	Hands, head, voice	Hands or arms > legs
Accompany-ing symptoms	None or symptoms of anxiety state	None	Rigidity, bradykinesia and postural instability
Frequency	10-14 Hz	7-10 Hz	3-7 Hz
Positional component	Posture > Kinetic	Posture > kinetic, may have a slight resting component if severe.	Resting, may have a postural and kinetic component in severe cases.
Symmetry	Bilateral, symmetric	Bilateral, can be mildly asymmetrical	Initially unilateral, bilateral and symmetrical in advanced stage
Course	Usually non progressive	Progressive	Progressive
Response to alcohol	Minimal or none	Responds significantly	None
Effect of caffeine, stress, stimulants	Increases	May increase	Increases with mental tasks
Inheritance	None	Autosomal dominant with variable penetrance	Sporadic or related to genetics of Parkinson's disease

Table 3.1 Comparison of Enhanced physiological, Essential and Parkinson's disease tremor.

Primary orthostatic tremor is usually a lower extremity tremor, which occurs upon standing and disappears with walking (involves the legs and trunk). This type of tremor has a very high frequency of 14 to 18 Hz, with bursts of motor unit activity. Upper limbs, if become involved in the tremor, are synchronous with the lower extremities. It may cause patients to feel unsteady while standing but not while walking except in severe cases. These patients do not have a problem sitting or lying down. The diagnosis of this tremor can be confirmed by electromyographic discharges of a 14-18 Hz pattern. All of the muscles in the legs, trunk and arm show this pattern, which is absent during sitting and lying down. Presence of a coherent high-frequency electromyographic discharge pattern, in all of the involved muscles, suggests that orthostatic tremor is a central tremor. This tremor can be treated with clonazepam, primidone and gabapentin although the response may not be great.

Primary writing tremor is characterized by its large amplitude and occurs at a frequency of 5-6 Hz. This tremor only occurs during the act of writing or when the hand assumes a writing position and only involves the affected arm. Primary writing tremor is often unilateral but may involve the other side in some advanced cases. This tremor may be difficult to distinguish from writer's cramp or essential tremor that is aggravated by writing. This type of tremor may respond to thalamic stimulation.

Cerebellar tremor causes a slow oscillation of approximately 3-5 Hz in a horizontal plane. Tremor of the head and trunk may be caused by midline cerebellar lesions. It is not a true tremor because in most cases it is ataxia of the affected limb or body part. It is important to distinguish this tremor from cerebellar outflow tremor. Cerebellar tremor does not respond to surgical treatments.

Dystonic Tremor is a postural and/or a kinetic tremor which is usually not seen during complete repose and occurs in a body part or limb affected by dystonia. These tremors are usually focal with irregular amplitudes and variable frequencies. Patients with cervical dystonia may have a head tremor and they may find that touching certain parts of their head or face with their hand or finger may help in transiently diminishing the amplitude of the tremor. This phenomenon is known as "sensory trick" and is helpful in establishing the diagnosis of dystonic head tremor.

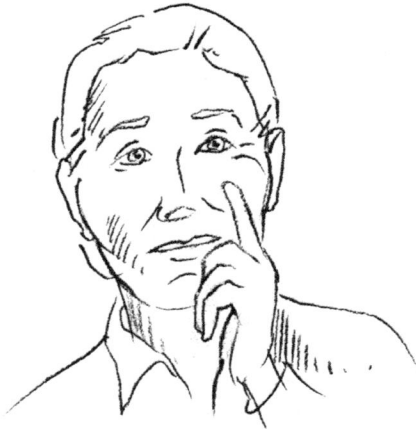

Figure 3.7 Dystonic head tremor stops by touching the side of face (sensory trick).

Patients with segmental dystonia may have both head and arm tremor. Postural hand tremor may be associated with cervical dystonia in about 30 percent of patients. Although this condition may become apparent at any age, symptoms usually begin between the ages of 20 to 60 years. Women are affected twice more than men.

Holme's tremor or midbrain tremor was first described by Gordon Holmes in 1904. It is an undulating tremor, present at rest but increases in severity through sustained posture of upper extremities and is further amplified during active movement. This tremor is characterized by a frequency of 2-5 Hz but has high amplitude and is extremely debilitating. The kinetic component is greater than postural component, and the postural component is greater than the resting component. This tremor is likely to be caused by interruption of fibers in the superior cerebellar peduncle which carry cerebello-thalamic and cerebello-olivary projections in the midbrain contralateral to the affected limb. Terms like rubral tremor or cerebellar outflow tremor have also been used for this type of tremor. Some of the known causes of midbrain tremor include cerebrovascular accidents, multiple sclerosis, infection, hypoxia, trauma, and cystic lesions which interrupt fibers of the superior cerebellar peduncle carrying cerebello-thalamic and cerebello-olivary projections in the midbrain. Ataxia and weakness may be accompanied features with Holmes tremors. Treatment of Holmes tremor is challenging as it responds poorly to medical treatments. There is only a partial response to pharmacological agents. Some evidence of partial improvement with anticholinergic therapy, dopaminergic agents alone or in combination with isoniazid is also found in literature. However, a significant response to stereotactic thalamatomy and DBS in ventralis intermedius nucleus of contralateral thalamus may be seen. As the treatment of midbrain tremor is difficult, surgery is an option early on in this condition. Botulinum toxin injections may help in dampening the amplitude of the tremor but may result in weakness of the affected hand and arm muscles. The effect of botulinum toxin lasts for about three to four months and the injections have to be repeated. In this type of tremor, treatment should be assessed on a case by case basis, and all options should be considered after a risk-benefit assessment.

Alcoholic tremor occurs in the lower body parts such as in the legs. It is usually 3 Hz in oscillation and can be differentiated from essential tremor by lack of family history of tremor and a greater responsiveness to propranolol.

Fragile X associated tremor-ataxia syndrome usually affects individuals above the age of 65 years. About two thirds of patients manifest a kinetic tremor. In fragile X syndrome A and fragile X-associated tremor-ataxia syndrome, there is expansion of CGG repeats of the FMR1 gene on chromosome Xq27.3. The normal number of CGG repeats is 6 to 50, the carriers have 50 to 200 repeats, and fragile X syndrome patients have 200 to 1500 repeats. About 1 in 1000 males and 1 in 250 females may carry the Fragile X Syndrome A premutation. The fragile X-associated tremor ataxia syndrome has a prevalence of 1 in 3000 men above age of 50. It is the most common form of X-linked mental retardation and there may be a family history of mental retardation. These patients have an IQ in the range of 25 to 70 with moderate to severe mental retardation. Mild intellectual deficit may be seen in about 30 to 50 percent of females with IQ in the range of 50 to 90. Males may have attention deficit hyperactivity disorder, anxiety, depression and autism. Seizures may be present in a minority of patients. During the early teen ages patients are noted to have macroorchidism, long face, prominent jaw, long and wide ears, and enlarged head. Elderly patients may have an impaired gait and fine motor skills, cerebellar ataxia, fluctuating weakness, sensory symptoms, sexual dysfunction, bladder or bowel dysfunction, parkinsonism, weakness of proximal lower extremities, and cognitive dysfunction. The patients with cognitive dysfunction have impaired executive functioning with relative sparing of language and visuospatial skills. Females with the premutation may have mild cognitive dysfunction with impairment of visual attention. In addition, females may have premature ovarian failure and early menopause. Females with fragile X-associated tremor/ataxia syndrome have also been described contrary to previous reports.

Psychogenic tremors have variable erratic frequency and fluctuations in amplitude. The tremor may go into remission for variable periods of time but may reoccur spontaneously. Usually the frequency is 6 Hz or less. The frequency of psychogenic tremor may correspond to the frequency of voluntary repetitive movements of the ipsilateral or contralateral limb. The patients may show an inability to perform the voluntary repetitive movements at a certain frequency requested by the examiner. However, the psychogenic tremor is a diagnosis of exclusion. If the abnormal movement is not rhythmical, the author prefers not to use the word tremor in the final diagnosis and rather describes the abnormal movement in detail.

The following features may be helpful in diagnosing psychogenic tremor:

1. Abrupt onset of symptoms.
2. Abnormal posture or movements disappearing with distraction.
3. Inconsistent movements or postures which change characteristics over time.
4. Incongruous movements and postures which do not fit with recognized physiological patterns.
5. Spontaneous remissions of symptoms.
6. Presence of additional abnormal movements inconsistent with the basic abnormal movement pattern or incongruous with a known movement disorder such as rhythmical shaking, slowness in carrying out voluntary movement and excessive startle in response to sudden, unexpected noise or threatening movement.
7. Presence of features of a paroxysmal disorder
8. Resolution of symptoms in response to placebo, suggestion or psychotherapy.

Medications induced tremors have an onset that is temporally related to the history of medication usage. The tremor is usually symmetrical and there may be more than one type of tremor present simultaneously.

Tardive tremor is seen in the context of long duration of use of antipsychotics. Dopamine antagonists and dopamine depleting drugs, especially with prolonged use, can cause tremor and parkinsonism with an incidence ranging from 10 to 60 percent depending on the type of drug used. However, in some cases the tremor and parkinsonism can even emerge within several days of treatment with these drugs. About 10 percent of patients may develop persistent and progressive tremors and parkinsonism despite the discontinuation of the causative drug. Females appear to have a higher incidence than males.

Following are the medications which have been implicated in the causation of drug induced tremors and parkinsonism:

A. Frequent causes of drug induced tremors and parkinsonsim:

1. Typical Antipsychotics:

    a. Phenothiazines: Chlorpromazine, triflupromazine, thioridazine, fluphenazine, piperazine, promethazine, prochlorperazine, perphenazine.

    b. Butyrophenones: Haloperidol, droperdol.

    c. Dibenzazepine: Loxapine.

    d. Diphenylbutylpiperidine: Pimozide

    e. Indolines: Molindone

    f. Substituted bezamides: Metoclopramide, cisapride, veralipride, alizapride, remoxipride, veralipride.

    g. Thioxanthenes: Chlorprothiexene, thiothixene.

2. Atypicals Antipsychotics:

Risperidone and olanzapine,

3. Dopamine depleting drugs:

Tetrabenzine and reserpine.

B. Infrequent causes of drug induced tremors and parkinsonism:

a. Anidepressants: SSRIs e.g., paroxetine, citalopram, fluoxetine and sertraline.
b. Immunosupressants: Cyclophosphamide, cytosine arabinoside, cyclosporine.
c. Mood stabilizers: Lithium and valproic acid.
d. Antihypertensives: Calcium channel blockers, diltiazem, nifedipine, verapamil, amlodipine, flunarizine, cinnarizine.
e. Other agents: Amphotericin B, amiodarone, meperidine, disulfiram, and methyldopa.

Lithium and valproic acid are associated with postural and kinetic tremor in many clinical settings.

INVESTIGATIONS:

In typical cases no investigations are required. When other alternative conditions are suspected the investigations may be directed to the possible underlying cause. The following investigations may be required in some cases:

TSH, serum glucose, electrolytes and CT scan of head if any focal or cerebellar signs are present. In young patients with suspicion of Wilson's disease, 24 hour urine copper, serum ceruloplasmin, serum copper and slit lamp examination for Kayser-Fleischer rings are required.

STAGING OF ESSENTIAL TREMOR:

Individual clinicians use different methods to grade the tremor and follow the progress in subsequent visits after the treatment is introduced. It is important to distinguish between the resting and action tremor since they are associated with different medical conditions. For resting tremor, the Unified Parkinson's Disease Rating Scale (UPDRS) may be used. The author finds the following simple scale for action tremor involving upper extremities, useful in the outpatient follow-up assessments.

A SCALE OF ACTION TREMOR:
(Devised by the author)

Grade 0 = No tremor on drawing a spiral of at least three circles without placing the hand on clipboard.

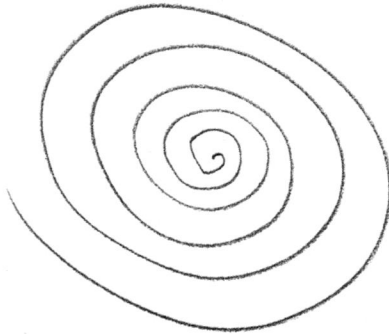

Figure 3.8 Normal Spiral

Grade 1 = Tremor present only on drawing a spiral of at least three circles without placing the hand on clipboard.

Grade 2 = Tremor present on writing a standard sentence with hand supported on the clipboard.

Grade 3 = Tremor causing spillage when a 4 inches tall glass, half filled with water, is moved from outstretched position to the mouth back and forth.

Grade 4 = Tremor causing spillage when a 4 inches tall glass, filled only one quarter or less with water, is moved from an outstretched position to the mouth back and forth.

The author finds the following simple scale for voice tremor helpful in the outpatient follow-up assessments.

A SCALE OF VOICE TREMOR:

(Devised by the author)

Grade 1: audible in sustained phonation (no aphonic breaks) but not in conversation.

Grade 2: audible in sustained phonation (no aphonic breaks) and in conversation (no aphonic breaks).

Grade 3: audible in sustained phonation (aphonic breaks) and in conversation (no aphonic breaks).

Grade 4: audible in sustained phonation (aphonic breaks) and in conversation (aphonic breaks).

REFERENCES:

Bain P, Brin M, Deuschl G, et al. Criteria for the diagnosis of essential tremor. Neurology 2000;54:67.

Bradley GW., Daroff R., Fenichel G., Marsden D. Neurology in Clinical Practice, Third edition. Butterworth & Heinmann, Woburn, MA 2000

Bukowczan S, Rudzińska M, Banach M, Szczudlik A. Holmes tremors is rare kind of tremors caused by lesion of rubro-spinal tract. Neuron Neurochir Pol. 2003;37 Suppl 5:83-8. Polish.

Elble RJ., Essential Tremor. Medlink. February 2007.

Gironell A, Kulisevsky J, Pascual-Sedano B, Barbanoj M. Routine neurophysiologic tremor analysis as a diagnostic tool for essential tremor: a prospective study. J Clin Neurophysiology 2004;21:446-50.

Goetz, CG. Textbook of Clinical Neurology, second edition, Saunders, Philadelphia, PA 2003

Hagerman RJ, Leavitt BR, Farzin F, et al. Fragile-X-associated tremor/ataxia syndrome (FXTAS) in females with the FMR1 premutation. Am J Hum Genet 2004;74:1051-6.

Hall DA, Berry-Kravis E, Jacquemont S, et al. Initial diagnoses given to persons with the fragile X associated tremor/ataxia syndrome (FXTAS). Neurology 2005;65:299-301.

Hertel F, Züchner M, Decker C, Erken E, Libri S, Schmitt M, Bettag M. Unilateral Holmes tremor, clearly responsive to cerebrospinal fluid release, in a patient with an ischemic midbrain lesion and associated chronic hydrocephalic ventricle enlargement. Case report. J Neurosurg. 2006 Mar; 104(3):448-51.

Inci S, Celik O, Soylemezoglu F, Ozgen T. Thalamomesencephalic ossified cavernoma presenting with Holmes' tremor. Surg Neurol. 2007 May;67(5):511-6; discussion 516.

Jacquemont S, Hagerman RJ, Leehey M, et al. Fragile X premutation tremor/ataxia syndrome: molecular, clinical, and neuroimaging correlates. Am J Hum Genetics 2003;72:869-78.

Jain S, Lo SE, Louis ED. Common misdiagnosis of a common neurological disorder: how are we misdiagnosing essential tremor? Archives of Neurology 2006;63:1100-4.

Jankovic J.,Tolosa E. Parkinson's Disease and Movement Disorder. Fifth edition, Lippincott Philadelphia, PA 2007

Klebe S, Stolze H, Grensing K, Volkmann J, Wenzelburger R, Deuschl G. Influence of alcohol on gait in patients with essential tremor. Neurology 2005;65(1):96-101.

Koster B, Lauk M, Timmer J, et al. Involvement of cranial muscles and high intermuscular coherence in orthostatic tremor. Ann Neurol 1999;45:384-8.

Louis ED, Ford B, Barnes LF. Clinical subtypes of essential tremor. Archives of Neurology 2000a;57(8):1194-8.

Louis ED, Ford B, Lee H, Andrews H, Camero G. Diagnostic criteria for essential tremor: a population perspective. Archives of Neurology 1998a;55:823-8.

Moller JC, Eggert KM, Unger M, Odin P, Chaudhuri KR, Oertei WH. Clinical risk–benefit assessment of dopamine agonists. European J of Neurology. 2008;15(2):15–23

Nikkhah G, Prokop T, Hellwig B, Lücking CH, Ostertag CB. Deep brain stimulation of the nucleus ventralis intermedius for Holmes (rubral) tremor and associated dystonia caused by upper brainstem lesions. Report of two cases. J Neurosurg. 2004;100(6):1079-83

Niranjan N Singh, Florian P Thomas, Fragile X-associated tremor/ataxia syndrome, MedLink, Aug 2008

Paulson GW. Benign essential tremor in childhood: symptoms, pathogenesis, treatment. Clin Pediatrics (Phila) 1976;15:67-70.

Paviour DC, Jäger HR, Wilkinson L, Jahanshahi M, Lees AJ. Holmes tremor: Application of modern neuroimaging techniques. Mov Disord. 2006 Dec; 21(12):2260-2.

Pezzini A, Zavarise P, Palvarini L, Viale P, Oladeji O, Padovani A. Holmes' tremor following midbrain Toxoplasma abscess: clinical features and treatment of a case. Parkinsonism Relat Disord. 2002 Jan;8(3):177-80.

Raethjen J, Kopper F, Govindan RB, Volkmann J, Deuschl G. Two different pathogenetic mechanisms in psychogenic tremor. Neurology 2004;63:812-5.

Ray L.W and Koller W.C. Movement Disorders, Neurologic Principles and Practice. Second edition. McGraw-Hill, USA, 2003.

Rivest J, Marsden CD. Trunk and head tremor as isolated manifestations of dystonia. Movement Disorders 1990;5:60-5.

Samie MR, Selhorst JB, Koller WC. Post-traumatic midbrain tremors. Neurology. 1990 Jan;40(1):62-6.

Sanborn MR, Danish SF, Ranaili NJ, Grady MS, Jaggi JL, Baltuch GH.Thalamic deep brain stimulation for midbrain tremor secondary to cystic degeneration of the brainstem. Stereotact Funct Neurosurg. 2009; 87(2):128-33. Epub 2009 Mar 6.

Sander HW, Masdeu JC, Tavoulareas G, Walters A, Zimmerman T, Chokroverty S. Orthostatic tremor: an electrophysiological analysis. Mov Disord 1998;13:735-8.

Schols L, Bauer P, Schmidt T, Schulte T, Riess O. Autosomal dominant cerebellar ataxias: clinical features, genetics, and pathogenesis. Lancet Neurol 2004;3:291-304.

Schrag A, Munchau A, Bhatia KP, Quinn NP, Marsden CD. Essential tremor: an overdiagnosed condition? J Neurol 2000;247:955-9.

Seidel S, Kasprian G, Leutmezer F, Prayer D, Auff. Disruption of nigrostriatal and cerebellothalamic pathways in dopamine responsive Holmes' tremor. J Neurol Neurosurg Psychiatry. 2009 Aug; 80(8):921-3. Epub 2008 May 1.

Shah M, Findley L, Muhammed N, Hawkes C. Olfaction is normal in essential tremor and can be used to distinguish it from Parkinson's disease. Movement Disorders 2005;20(Suppl 10):S166.

Slawek J, Szymkiewicz-Rogowska A, Friedman A. Rubral tremor of Holmes, rare case of pathological tremor: case report. Neurol Neurochir Pol. 2000 Jul-Aug;34(4):775-82. Polish.

Soland VL, Bhatia KP, Volonte MA, Marsden CD. Focal task-specific tremors. Movement Disorders 1996;11:665-70.

Abdul Qayyum Rana, MD, FRCPC

Walker M, Kim H, Samii A. Holmes-like tremors of the lower extremity following brainstem hemorrhage. Mov Disord. 2007 Jan 15; 22(2):272-4.

Chapter 4

TREATMENT OF ESSENTIAL TREMOR

A. MEDICAL TREAMTMENT:

Sometimes patients with essential tremor may desire nothing more than to be assured that they don't have Parkinson's disease. Any exacerbating factors, if present, should be addressed first. The avoidance of stimulants such as caffeine is helpful in some cases. If the tremor does not affect daily functioning it could be observed. Milder cases of essential tremor may be helped with occupational therapy training or use of weighted wrist bracelets that are available at many sports stores.

Alcohol may transiently reduce tremor amplitude in about 50 to 90 percent of the cases, but the rebound tremor may be worse when the effect of alcohol wears off. Alcohol intake is not recommended for treatment of essential tremor.

Cooling the upper limbs in cold water for about 5 minutes causes temporary reduction in essential tremor. Essential tremor is also suppressed by general anesthesia.

The most commonly used medications are propranolol, a beta-blocker and primidone, a GABA agonist.

i) BETA BLOCKERS

Among the beta-blockers, the most effective medication is *Propranolol*. Propranolol use for essential tremor was introduced in 1971. Among the different beta-blockers, none is considered to be superior to propranolol. Drugs that are predominantly *B-1* antagonists are less effective than those that act on *B-2* receptors as well. Overall, about 25 percent of patients are able to maintain their initial improvement for about 2 years. It is a nonselective beta-adrenergic receptor antagonist. Some patients may take propranolol only before social engagements whereas others may use it on a daily basis. If propranolol is to be taken on daily basis, the dosage ranges from 60 mg to 260 mg per day. Propranolol is effective in treating essential tremor involving limbs, and many studies have shown that the magnitude of tremor is reduced by at least 50 percent as measured by accelerometry and clinical rating scale.

Side effects include a drop in blood pressure, fatigue, depression, impotence and bradycardia. Propranolol is contraindicated in patients with asthma, COPD or heart failure. Diabetes mellitus is also a relative contraindication as propranolol can mask symptoms of hypoglycemia.

Propranolol LA may be taken only once a day as it is a long acting preparation. Propanolol LA is also effective in improving limb tremor. In one study Propranolol LA caused about 30-38% improvement in limb tremor when measured by accelerometry. Propranolol, propranolol LA and primidone exhibit a similar therapeutic effect for the limb tremor.

Atenolol also has a positive therapeutic effect on limb tremor. The dose is 50-150 mg per day. About 25 percent mean improvement on the clinical rating scale and a 37 percent improvement by accelerometry were noticed in one study. However, side effects such as lightheadedness, nausea, cough, dry mouth and sleepiness may limit its use.

In one study, *Nadolol,* at a dose of 120-240 mg daily, resulted in about 60-70 percent improvement by accelerometry in patients who previously responded to propranolol. The side effects include dizziness.

ii) PRIMIDONE

Primidone, conventionally used as an antiepileptic medication, provides a significant therapeutic benefit for essential tremor It is a GABA agonist. The initial dose is one quarter of a tablet of 125 mg (31.25 mg) which is increased slowly. The average reduction in tremor is at least 50 percent when measured by the clinical rating scale and accelerometry. One third of the patients may have a strong feeling of being unwell and experience side effects of drowsiness, confusion, nausea, and dizziness upon the initiation of this drug. However, these side effects may improve in 2 to 3 weeks time.

Combined treatment with propranolol and primidone is more effective than monotherapy with either of these agents alone. In one study, the addition of 50-1000 mg/day of primidone to propranolol reduced the tremor amplitude more than when propranolol was used alone. Propranolol at an average dosage of 260 mg/day (its maximum effective dosage) reduced tremor amplitude by a mean of 35 percent, but the addition of primidone (50-1000 mg/day) decreased the tremor amplitude by a mean of 60 – 70 percent.

Propranolol and primidone alone are almost equally effective in the treatment of both postural and kinetic tremor, but the combination of these two drugs is more effective than either drug used alone. The combined treatment with primidone and propranolol can be used to treat limb tremor when monotherapy is not sufficient. The theraputic effects of primidone and propranolol on postural and kinetic tremor last for at least several years. However, the response may decrease partially with time. The dosage of primidone and propranolol may need to be increased with time.

iii) OTHER THERAPIES.

Topiramate is a sodium channel blocker. Its common indications include epilepsy and prophylaxis of migraine. It has a mild to moderate effect in reducing essential tremor. In one study, it resulted in about a 22-37 percent mean improvement in limb tremor when measured by the clinical rating scale. The initial starting dose of topiramate is 25 mg once a day, a dosage which is increased slowly to two or three times daily.

Side effects include decrease in appetite, weight loss, paresthesias, concentration difficulties, exacerbation of glaucoma and renal stone.

Gabapentin has a mild to moderate beneficial effect on essential tremor. In one study, gabapentin reduced postural and kinetic tremor when administered at a dose of 1200 mg/day. When gabapentin was used as a monotherapy, there was about a 77 percent improvement by accelerometry and a 33 percent improvement on the clinical rating scale. The side effects include fatigue, dizziness, nervousness and lethargy.

In one study, benzodiazepines, especially *clonazepam,* significantly reduced the kinetic tremor. There was about a 71 percent mean improvement by accelerometry and a 26-57 percent improvement in limb tremor on the clinical rating scale. The dose ranged from 0.5 to 6 mg/day. Side effects include drowsiness. There is a potential of abuse and possibility of withdrawal symptoms associated with clonazepam, and therefore it should be used with a great caution.

Nimodipine may significantly reduce the amplitude of limb tremor. The usual dose is 30 mg four times daily. About 53 percent improvement by accelerometry and a 45 percent improvement on the clinical rating scale were noticed in one study. The side effects include headache and heartburn.

Alprazolam has also shown some beneficial effects on limb tremor. In one study, when compared to a placebo, a 25-35 percent improvement in limb tremor was noticed. Use of alprazolam is cautioned due to its abusive potential. Side effects include lightheadedness, nausea, cough, dry mouth and sleepiness.

Treatment of limb tremor with atenolol, topiramate, and gabapentin is not as effective as propanolol or primidone. Therefore, atenolol, topiramate, and gabapentin are considered for treatment of postural and kinetic limb tremor if propanolol or primidone are not helpful.

Nimodipine may be considered for the treatment of essential tremor affecting limbs, when other agents are not helpful.

Botulinum toxin may offer some improvement but may cause finger or wrist weakness. Botulinum toxin has been used to treat hand, head and voice tremor variants of the essential tremor syndrome. About a 67 percent improvement in head tremor was noticed by accelerometry in one study. The side effects include pain at the injection site and weakness. The effect of botulinum toxin on essential tremor affecting limbs is mild. About a 20 percent improvement in postural tremor and a 27 percent improvement in kinetic tremor were noticed in one study. It may reduce head and voice tremor, but when used to treat voice tremor, botulinum toxin may cause hoarseness of voice and swallowing difficulties. In one study, about a 22 percent improvement with unilateral injections and a 30 percent improvement with bilateral injections were noticed in voice tremor. The botulinum toxin injections for limb, head and voice tremor may be considered in medically refractory cases.

Drug	Dose	Side effects	Comments
Primidone	Starting dose is 31.25 mg once daily, increased slowly up to 250 mg three times daily	Sedation, fatigue, drowsiness, nausea, vomiting, malaise and dizziness.	GABA agonist.
Propranolol	Starting dose is 40 mg twice daily, increased slowly up to 180 mg twice daily	Lightheadedness, bradycardia, drowsiness, impotence, fatigue, depression.	*B1 & B2* antagonist.
Propranolol LA	Starting dose is 80 mg once daily, increased slowly up to 320 mg/day	Skin rash, lightheadedness and dizziness	Same as propranolol but long acting.
Topiramate	Starting dose is 25 mg once daily, increased weekly by 50 mg/day to the maximum dose of 200 mg twice daily	Weight loss, paresthesias, concentration difficulties, exacerbation of glaucoma and renal stones.	Sodium channel blocker.
Gabapentin	Starting dose is 300 mg once daily, increased over few days to 300- 900 mg three times daily	Fatigue, dizziness, nervousness, lethargy	Alpha-2-delta calcium channel subunit blocker.
Nadolol	Starting dose is 40 mg once daily. maximum 240 mg/day	Dizziness	*B1 & B2* antagonist.
Atenolol	Starting dose is 50 mg once daily, maximum 150 mg/day	Lightheadedness, nausea, cough, dry mouth, sleepiness.	*B1* antagonist.
Clonazepam	Starting dose is 0.5 mg once daily, increased slowly to 2 mg three times daily	Lethargy	Benzodiazepine.
Nimodipine	Starting dose is 30 mg once daily, increased slowly to maximum 120 mg/day divided three times daily	Headaches and heartburn	Ca channel blocker
Alprazolam	Starting dose is 0.25 mg three times daily, increased slowly up to 1 mg three times daily	Fatigue, drowsiness, abuse potential	Benzodiazepine

Drug	Dose	Side effects	Comments
Botulinum toxin A for head tremor	Dose ranges from 50 to 400 units depending upon the muscles involved and degree of tremor.	Excessive weakness of injected muscles, dysphagia, injection pain.	Injected every 3-4 months.
Botulinum toxin A for hand tremor	Dose is variable, from 50-100 Units/arm	Hand and finger weakness, pain at injection site.	Injected every 3-4 months.
Botulinum toxin A for voice tremor	0.5-15 Units	Hypophonia, dysphagia	Injected every 3-4 months.

Table 4.1: Pharmacological agents used
in the treatment of Essential tremor.

Order of Preference	Drugs
First Choice	Propranolol, Primidone, or the combination of these two agents.
Second Choice	Topiramate, Atenolol, Gabapentin, Clonazepam
Third Choice	Alprazolam, Clozapine, Nadolol, Nimodipine.

Table 4.2 Choices of medical treatments used
for Essential tremor affecting Limbs.

B. SURGICAL TREATMENTS:

Surgical treatments are used for patients who have very advanced essential tremor which is refractory to the pharmacological management. Two types of surgical treatments are done; *thalamotomy* and *deep brain thalamic stimulation.*

Surgical procedures such as stimulation of the nucleus ventralis intermedius or ablation are used for intractable tremor, and a significant improvement in the tremor has been reported. In presurgical assessment, patients are evaluated by a multidisciplinary team, including a neurologist with expertise in movement disorders, a neurosurgeon and a neuropsychologist. Appropriate brain imaging is also performed. The procedure may be unilateral or bilateral depending on the degree of tremor.

1. Unilateral deep brain stimulation results in marked improvement of contralateral postural and kinetic tremor. In one study, about a 60-90 percent improvement on the clinical rating scale was noticed in limb tremor. Voice tremor usually does not improve by the unilateral nucleus ventralis intermedius stimulation. Inconsistent results have been reported about the response of head tremor to unilateral or bilateral deep brain stimulation. Deep brain stimulation has shown greater improvement and fewer side effects than thalamotomy. However, these procedures are invasive and side effects like speech and swallowing problems, sensory disturbances and balance problems may occur. There is also a risk of infection and hemorrhage associated with these procedures. The side effects of this treatment can usually be reduced by adjusting the stimulus parameters, but this may result in reduced tremor suppression and efficacy.

2. Unilateral thalamotomy is very effective for the treatment of contralateral limb tremor, while bilateral thalamotomy has frequent and severe side effects. In one study, about a 55-90 percent improvement on the clinical rating scale was noticed. Relief of essential tremor after thalamotomy has been thought to be related to disruption of abnormal thalamocortical synchronization. The first thalamotomy for essential tremor was performed in the early 1960s.

Gamma knife thalamotomy is performed by delivering radiation to an intracranial target determined by brain imaging. In one study, there was about a 70-80 percent improvement seen on the clinical rating scale, however, some delayed complications have been reported with this technique. Although good results have been reported in several studies, the evidence is insufficient to recommend this treatment for essential tremor.

Technique	Side effects	Comments
Deep brain thalamic stimulation	Dysarthria, weakness, numbness, headache, intracranial hemorrhage, dysequilibrium and decreased verbal fluency.	Marked improvement in limb tremor, insufficient evidence for voice and head tremor, side effects are less than thalamotomy.
Thalamotomy	Transient contralateral weakness, dysarthria, contralateral hemiparesis, verbal or cognitive deficits and confusion.	Marked improvement of contralateral tremor. Side effects more with bilateral procedure

Gamma knife Thalamotomy	Transient contralateral arm weakness and numbness, dysarthria, dystonia of the contralateral arm and leg.	Insufficient evidence.

Table 4.3: Surgical treatments of Essential Tremor.

PROGNOSIS:

Essential tremor is a lifelong disorder that gradually worsens with advancing age. The life span and the general health of the patient are not affected. This condition causes significant interference with employment, daily activities and social functioning.

REFERENCES:

Benabid AL, Pollak P, Gao D, et al. Chronic electrical stimulation of the ventralis intermedius nucleus of the thalamus as a treatment of movement disorders. J Neurosurg 1996;84(2):203-14.

Bradley GW., Daroff R., Fenichel G., Marsden D. Neurology in Clinical Practice, Third edition. Butterworth & Heinmann, Woburn, MA 2000

Elble RJ. Essential Tremor. Medlink. February 2007.

Goetz, CG. Textbook of Clinical Neurology. Second edition, Saunders, Philadelphia, PA 2003

Jankovic J.,Tolosa E. Parkinson's Disease and Movement Disorder. Fifth edition, Lippincott Philadelphia, PA 2007

Kumar R, Lozano AM, Sime E, Lang AE. Long-term follow-up of thalamic deep brain stimulation for essential and parkinsonian tremor. Neurology 2003;61:1601-4.

Murata J, Kitagawa M, Uesugi H, et al. Electrical stimulation of the posterior subthalamic area for the treatment of intractable proximal tremor. J Neurosurg 2003;99:708-15

Obwegeser AA, Uitti RJ, Turk MF, Strongosky AJ, Wharen RE. Thalamic stimulation for the treatment of midline tremors in essential tremor patients. Neurology 2000;54:2342-4.

Ohye C, Shibazaki T, Zhang J, Andou Y. Thalamic lesions produced by gamma thalamotomy for movement disorders. J Neurosurg 2002;97(5 Suppl):600-6.

Ondo WG, Jankovic J, Connor GS, et al. Topiramate in essential tremor: a double-blind, placebo-controlled trial. Neurology 2006;66:672-7.

Pahapill PA, Levy R, Dostrovsky JO, et al. Tremor arrest with thalamic microinjections of muscimol in patients with essential tremor. Annals of Neurology 1999;46:249-52.

Papavassiliou E, Rau G, Heath S, et al. Thalamic deep brain stimulation for essential tremor: relation of lead location to outcome. Neurosurgery 2004;54:1120-30.

Paulson GW. Benign essential tremor in childhood: symptoms, pathogenesis, treatment. Clin Pediatrics (Phila) 1976;15:67-70.

Plaha P., Patel NK, Gill SS. Stimulation of the subthalamic region for essential tremor. J Neurosurg 2004;101:48-54.

Ray L.W and Koller W.C. Movement Disorders, Neurologic Principles and Practice. Second edition. McGraw-Hill, USA. 2003.

Schuurman PR, Bosch DA, Bossuyt PM, et al. A comparison of continuous thalamic stimulation and thalamotomy for suppression of severe tremor. New England Journal of Medicine 2000;342:461-8.

Siderowf A. Gollump SM, Stern MB, Baltuch GH, Riina HA. Emergence of complex, involuntary movements after gamma knife radiosurgery for essential tremor. Movement Disorders 2001;16:965-7.

Stover NP, Okun MS, Evatt ML, Raju DV, Bakay RA, Vitek JL. Stimulation of the subthalamic nucleus in a patient with Parkinson disease and essential tremor. Archives of Neurology 2005;62:141-3.

Sydow O, Thobois S, Alesch F, Speelman JD. Multicentre European study of thalamic stimulation in essential tremor: a six year follow up. Journal of Neurology, Neurosurgery, Psychiatry 2003;74:1387-91.

Taha JM, Janszen MA, Favre J. Thalamic deep brain stimulation for the treatment of head, voice, and bilateral limb tremor. J Neurosurg 1999;91:68-72.

Ushe M, Mink JW, Revilla FJ, et al. Effect of stimulation frequency on tremor suppression in essential tremor. Movement Disorders 2004;19:1163-8.

Zackowski KM, Bastian AJ, Hakimian S, et al. Thalamic stimulation reduces essential tremor but not the delayed antagonist muscle timing. Neurology 2002;58:402-10.

Zesiewicz TA, Elble R, Louis ED, et al. Practice parameter: therapies for essential tremor: report of the Quality Standards Subcommittee of the American Academy of Neurology. Neurology 2005;64:2008-20.

Chapter 5

SAMPLE CASES

CASE NO 1.

I.D. Mr. D.G. is an 18 year old right handed male.

Chief complaint: Tremor of hands

History of present illness: This patient initially noticed tremor of his right hand three months ago and recently started noticing a slight tremor of his left hand as well. The tremor usually occurs when he is holding objects such as a cup of coffee and during activity. There is no tremor when his hands are in a resting position. There has been no change in his handwriting. He has no problem in writing, drinking from a glass full of liquids, eating, or carrying out other activities of daily life. He does not drink alcohol. He has no history of thyroid disease, use of antipsychotics or exposure to any toxins. The rest of the neurological inquiry was normal.

Past medical history: Non contributory

Medications: None

Social history: He does not smoke. He is a student.

Family history: His father has a similar tremor.

Review of system: Unremarkable

Physical Examination: He had a mild amplitude, 9 HZ, flexion-extension tremor of both hands when outstretched, in wing beating position and on finger-nose-finger testing without any intention component. There was no resting tremor, bradykinesia or rigidity. There was no tremor of his voice, head, lips, chin, jaw, or lower extremities. The rest of the neurological examination, including tandem gait, was normal. His handwriting did not show any tremor. Spiral drawing showed a minimal tremor.

Diagnosis: Essential tremor. The tremor is not interfering with activities of daily life.

Treatment: Observation.

CASE NO 2.

I.D. Mr. B.M. is a 75 year old right handed male.

Chief complaint: Tremor of both hands

History of present illness: About two years ago, this patient noticed tremor of both of his hands that has worsened over the last 6 months. The onset was gradual. The tremor occurs when he is holding objects such as a glass of water, during activity as well as when his hands are in a resting position. His handwriting has become very course over the last year. He finds difficulty in drinking fluids, pouring, and using a spoon and fork while eating. He has stopped eating out because of embarrassment. He is slightly slow in walking, a result that he attributes to arthritis; he may occasionally drool at night time while sleeping. His balance is not as great as it was before, and he may feel unsteady on his feet when he turns quickly. However, this has not resulted in any falls. He does not drink alcohol. He has no history of thyroid disease. There is no history of use of antipsychotics or exposure to any toxins. The rest of the neurological inquiry was normal.

Past medical history: Hypertension

Medications: Ramipril 5 mg once daily.

Social history: He does not smoke or drink, he is a retired driver.

Family history: Unremarkable

Review of system: Unremarkable

Physical examination: He had moderate amplitude, 8 HZ, flexion extension tremor of both hands when outstretched, in wing beating position and on finger-nose-finger testing without any intention component. There was a mild amplitude, 8 HZ, flexion extension, resting tremor of both hands which disappeared on complete repose in supine position, and a mild amplitude tremor of voice audible on sustained phonation (no aphonic breaks). There was no tremor of head, lips, chin, jaw or lower extremities. He had mild cogwheeling of both upper extremities at the elbows. There was no bradykinesia. His speed of waking was slightly slow, his gait was of an antalgic pattern. The rest of the neurological examination including tandem gait was normal. His handwriting and spiral drawing showed a moderate kinetic tremor.

Diagnosis: Essential tremor interfering with activities of daily life.

Treatment: Propranolol

CASE NO 3

I.D. Mrs. A.K. is a 57 year old right handed female.

Chief complaint: Head tremor

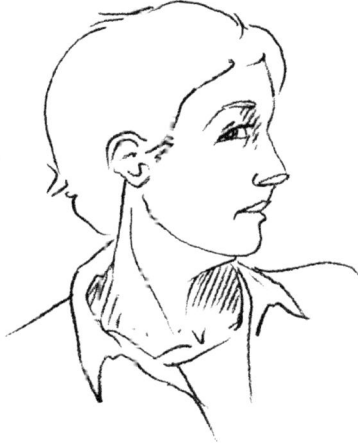

Figure 5.1 Patient with head tremor

History of present illness: This patient initially noticed a head tremor nine months ago. She reports that her head shakes side to side and tends to go towards the left side on its own. While driving and watching TV she feels that her head is being pulled to the left side. By touching the side of her face she can bring her head back to a neutral position ceasing the tremor. However, as soon as she removes her hand, the head tilts back to the left side. The tremor is interfering with her social and household activities. She has a constant neck pain as well. There is no tremor involving her hands, lips, jaw, chin or legs. She denies any change in her handwriting. She does not drink alcohol. There is no history of use of antipsychotics or exposure to any toxins. She has no known history of thyroid disease. The rest of the neurological inquiry was normal.

Past medical history: Hypertension

Medications: Atenolol 50 mg daily.

Social history: She does not smoke or drink, she is a housewife.

Family history: Unremarkable

Review of system: Unremarkable

Physical examination: There was a 30 degree turn of her head towards the left side. There was a mildly decreased range of motion of her neck to the right side. She had a mild amplitude, 5 HZ, side to side (NO- NO) tremor of her head. There was no shift of her head. The right sternocleidomastoid muscle was mildly hypertrophied when compared to the left side. She was able to bring her head to a neutral position solely by touching the side of her head. Her left shoulder was higher and slightly anteriorly displaced. There was no tremor of her hands or upper extremities. There was no tremor of voice, lips, chin, jaw or lower extremities. The rest of the neurological examination, including tandem gait, was normal. Her handwriting and spiral drawing did not reveal any tremor.

Diagnosis: Dystonic head tremor.

Treatment: Botulinum toxin, 25 units were injected at two sites in the right sternocleidomastoid muscle and 25 units were injected at two sites in the left levator scapulae muscle. She had a significant relief of her head tremor few weeks later.

CASE NO 4.

I.D. Mr. D.G. is a 48 year old right handed male.

Chief complaint: Hand tremor

History of present illness: This patient initially noticed tremor of both of his hands about six months ago. The tremor occurs mainly when he is holding objects and during activity. There is no tremor when his hands are in a resting position. His handwriting has become very course overtime. His tremor is particularly worse in the morning after he wakes up. He has significant problem in writing, drinking fluids from a glass, eating, and carrying out other daily activities. He does not drink alcohol. He has no history of thyroid disease. There is no history of the use of antipsychotics or exposure to any toxins. The rest of the neurological inquiry was normal.

Past medical history: Migraine

Medications: Amitryptaline 20 mg once daily.

Social history: He does not smoke. He is an engineer.

Family history: Unremarkable

Review of system: Unremarkable

Physical Examination: He had a moderate amplitude, 8 HZ, flexion extension tremor of both hands when outstretched, in a wing beating position and on finger-nose-finger testing without any intention component.

There was no resting tremor. There was no tremor of his voice, head, lips, chin, jaw, or lower extremities. The rest of the neurological examination, including tandem gait, was normal. His handwriting and spiral drawing showed a moderate tremor.

Diagnosis: Essential tremor.

Treatment: He was started on propranolol 40 mg twice daily, which helped his tremor significantly. With propranolol, his headaches also improved. He was able to stop amitryptaline without any further worsening of his headaches.

CASE NO 5

I.D. Mrs. A.K. is a 59 year old right handed female.

Chief complaint: Head tremor

History of present illness: This patient initially noticed tremor of her head about nine months ago. She reports that her head shakes from side to side. There is no history of head turning or pulling to any side. There is no improvement in her head tremor upon touching the side of her face or head. However, she did notice that her head tremor improves with alcohol intake. There is no history of neck pain. The head tremor is significantly interfering with social and household activities. Her friends have also commented on her head tremor. There is no tremor of her hands, arms, lips, jaw, chin or legs. She denies any change in her handwriting. There is no history of the use of antipsychotics or exposure to any toxins. She has no history of thyroid disease. The rest of the neurological inquiry was normal.

Past medical history: COPD

Medications: Atrovent ® and ventoline ® inhalers PRN

Family history: Her father had a tremor of hands on holding things.

Social history: She does not smoke. She is a housewife.

Review of system: Unremarkable

Physical examination: She had a mild amplitude, 7 HZ, side to side (NO- NO) tremor of her head, there was no turn, tilt or shift of her head. There was no asymmetry in the size of her head and neck muscles. There was no tremor of her hands or upper extremities in the outstretched or wing beating position, on the finger-nose-finger testing or at rest. There was no tremor of voice, lips, chin, jaw or lower extremities. The rest of the neurological examination, including tandem gait, was normal. Her handwriting and spiral drawing did not reveal any tremor.

Diagnosis: Isolated head tremor, an essential tremor variant.

Treatment: Propranolol was contraindicated because of COPD. She was started on primidone 31.25 mg daily, she reported about a 20 % improvement in her head tremor. The dose was increased to 62.5 mg on the next visit, but upon increasing the dose she became severely dizzy and stopped taking primidone. She did not want to take oral medications any more. She wanted to try Botulinum toxin. She was injected 25 units of Botulinum toxin at two sites in the sternocleidomastoid muscle on each side. She had a moderate relief of her head tremor. The dose was increased to 25 units at three sites in each sternocleidomastoid which resulted in further relief of her head tremor.

CASE NO 6

I.D. Mr. L.D is a 47 year old right handed male.

Chief complaint: Hand tremor

History of present illness: This patient noticed tremor of his both hands about a year ago, but recently he has noticed a significant worsening of his tremor. The tremor occurs mainly on holding objects and during activity. There is no tremor when his hands are in the resting position. His handwriting has become very course. He has difficulty in writing, drinking fluids from a glass, eating, or carrying out other activities of daily life. He does not drink alcohol. He has no history of thyroid disease. He has no history of use of antipsychotics, or exposure to any toxins. The rest of the neurological inquiry was normal.

Past medical history: Diabetes mellitus. He has history of several hypoglycaemic episodes in the past.

Medications: Metformin® 500 mg BID, Lipitor® 20 mg once daily

Social history: He does not smoke. He is the superintendent of an apartment building.

Family history: His father had a similar tremor

Review of system: Unremarkable

Physical Examination: He had a moderate amplitude, 8 HZ, flexion extension tremor of both of his hands when outstretched, in the wing beating position and on finger-nose-finger testing without any intention component. There was no resting tremor. There was no tremor of his voice, head, lips, chin, jaw, or lower extremities. The rest of the neurological examination, including tandem gait, was normal. His handwriting and spiral drawing showed significant tremor.

Diagnosis: Essential tremor.

Treatment: Propranolol was contraindicated because of the history of hypoglycemic episodes. He was started on primidone 31.25 mg once daily. He reported a mild improvement of his tremor. Upon increasing the dose to 62.5 mg and then to 125 mg of primidone, he continued experiencing significant benefit.

CASE NO 7

I.D. Mr. J. M. is a 64 year old right handed male.

Chief complaint: Hand tremor

History of present illness: This patient initially noticed tremor of his right hand about 2 months ago, but recently he has noticed a further worsening of his tremor. The tremor is present only when his hands are in the resting position and disappears when he uses his hands. His handwriting has become small, but he has no difficulty in drinking fluids from a glass, eating, or carrying out other daily activities. He does not drink alcohol. He has no history of the use of antipsychotics or exposure to any toxins. The rest of the neurological inquiry was unremarkable.

Past medical history: Hypertension.

Medications: Ramipril 5 mg daily

Social history: He does not smoke. He is an accountant.

Family history: His mother had Parkinson's disease.

Review of system: Unremarkable

Physical Examination: He had a mild amplitude, 5 HZ, supination, pronation, resting tremor of the right hand, but no tremor when his hands were outstretched, in the wing beating position or on the finger-nose-finger testing. There was no tremor of voice, head, lips, chin, jaw, or lower extremities. There was no rigidity or bradykinesia. The rest of the neurological examination, including tandem gait, was normal except that his tremor got worse when he was walking. His handwriting was very small in size.

Diagnosis: Resting tremor of Parkinson's disease.

Treatment: Amantadine 100 mg three times daily. He had significant improvement of his tremor with amantadine.

CASE NO 8

I.D. Mr. S. M. is a 38 year old right handed male.

Chief complaint: Hand tremor

History of present illness: This patient initially noticed tremor of both of his hands about 1 ½ year ago. The tremor occurs mainly when he is holding objects and during activity. There is no tremor when his hands are in the resting position. His handwriting has become very course. He has difficulty in writing, drinking fluids from a glass, eating, or carrying out other activities of daily life. He does not drink alcohol. He has no history of thyroid disease. He has been on valproic acid for bipolar disorder for the last two years and is currently stable. He has no history of exposure to any toxins. The rest of the neurological inquiry was unremarkable.

Past medical history: Bipolar disorder.

Medications: Valproic acid 250 mg TID

Social history: He does not smoke. He is currently on disability.

Family history: Unremarkable

Review of system: Unremarkable

Physical Examination: He had a moderate amplitude, 8 HZ, flexion extension tremor of both hands when outstretched, in the wing beating position, and on the finger-nose-finger testing without any intention component. There was a very mild amplitude, 8 HZ, flexion extension tremor of both hands in the resting position. There was no tremor of his voice, head, lips, chin, jaw, or lower extremities. There was no rigidity or bradykinesia. The rest of the neurological examination, including tandem gait, was normal. His handwriting and spiral drawing showed moderate tremor. There was no micrographia on handwriting.

Diagnosis: Postural, kinetic and resting tremor of both upper extremities likely induced by valproic acid. The tremor is interfering with his daily activities.

Treatment: Suggestions were made to his psychiatrist to change valproic acid to another mood stabilizer which would not exacerbate the tremor.

CASE NO 9

I.D. Mr. R.P. is a 41 year old right handed male.

Chief complaint: Hand tremor

History of present illness: This patient initially noticed tremor of both of his hands about one year ago. There has been no worsening of his tremor over time. The tremor is present in both of his hands while in the resting position, holding objects and during activity. His handwriting has become very course. He has difficulty in writing, drinking fluids from a glass, eating, or carrying out other daily activities. He does not drink alcohol. He has no history of thyroid disease. He has been on risperidone for psychotic depression for the last 1 ½ year, and is currently stable. He has no history of exposure to any toxins. The rest of the neurological inquiry was normal.

Past medical history: Psychotic depression.

Medications: Risperidone 2 mg BID

Social history: He does not smoke. He is on disability. He was an accountant.

Family history: Unremarkable

Review of system: Unremarkable

Physical Examination: He had a moderate amplitude, 8 HZ, flexion extension tremor of both hands in the resting position, while outstretched, in the wing beating position and on the finger-nose-finger testing without any intention component. There was no tremor of voice, head, lips, chin, jaw, or lower extremities. He had mild cogwheeling of both upper extremities. There was no rigidity or bradykinesia. The rest of the neurological examination, including gait, was normal. His handwriting and spiral drawing showed significant tremor.

Diagnosis: Tremor of both upper extremities likely induced by risperidone. The tremor is interfering with his daily activities.

Treatment: Suggestions were made to his psychiatrist to change risperidone to another antipsychotic with a better side effect profile. Risperidone was changed to quetiapine by his psychiatrist. He was seen 6 months later and his tremor had significantly improved.

CASE NO 10

I.D. Mr. D.C. is a 28 year old right handed male.

Chief complaint: Tremor of hands

History of present illness: This patient initially noticed tremor of both of his hands three months ago. The tremor occurs mainly while holding objects and during activity. There is no tremor when his hands are in the resting position. There is no significant change in his handwriting. He has no problem in writing, drinking fluids from a glass, eating, or carrying out other daily activities. He does not drink alcohol. He has history of poor heat tolerance, increased perspiration, diarrhoea, palpitation, and increased appetite. He has no history of the use of antipsychotics or exposure to any toxins. The rest of the neurological inquiry was normal.

Past medical history: Non contributory

Medications: None

Social history: He does not smoke. He is a student.

Family history: Unremarkable

Review of system: Unremarkable

Physical Examination: He had a mild amplitude, 12 HZ, flexion extension tremor of both hands when outstretched. There was no tremor in the wing beating position and on the finger-nose-finger testing. There was no resting tremor and no tremor of voice, head, lips, chin, jaw, or lower extremities. The rest of the neurological examination, including tandem gait, was normal. His resting pulse rate was 105. His handwriting and spiral drawing did not reveal any tremor.

Investigations: Serum TSH was much below the normal range with increase in T4 and T3 level.

Diagnosis: Tremor likely due to hyperthyroidism.

Treatment: A referral to endocrinology service was made.

INDEX

A

Action Tremor 7
Alcoholic Tremor 9, 44
Alprazolam 61, 63, 64
Atenolol 59, 63, 64, 76

B

Beta Blockers 58
Botulinum Toxin 20, 44, 62

C

Cerebellar Tremor 5, 8, 9,
    41, 42
Classification of Tremor 4
Clonazepam 41, 61
Course of Essential Tremor 12
Criteria for the Diagnosis of
    Essential Tremor 34

D

Deep Brain Stimulation 54,
    65
Diagnosis of Essential Tremor
    28, 34
Drug induced Tremors and
    Parkinsonism 47, 48
Dysdiadokinesia 34
Dystonic Tremor 5, 9

E

Enhanced Physiological
    Tremor 5, 7, 9
Epidemiology of Essential
    Tremor 11
Etiology and Pathogenesis of
    Essential Tremor 13
Exacerbating Factors for
    Essential Tremor 13,
    57

F

Finger-Nose-Finger Testing
    31, 72, 74, 78, 81, 83,
    84, 86, 89, 90
Fragile X Tremor-Ataxia Syn-
    drome 44
Frequencies of Different
    Tremor syndromes 9

G

Gabapentin 41, 61, 62
Gamma Knife Thalamotomy
    66
Glass Test 31

H

Heel-Knee-Shin Testing 34
Holme's Tremor 43

Printed in Great Britain
by Amazon